Conquering Stress and Despair: A Comprehensive Guide to Managing and Overcoming Difficult Emotions

By Fredrick G

Table of Contents

I. Introduction

1. The Purpose of This Book
2. What You Can Expect to Learn
3. The Impact of Stress and Despair

II. Understanding Stress and Despair

1. What is Stress?
2. Common Causes of Stress
3. The Effects of Stress on the Body and Mind
4. What is Despair?
5. Common Causes of Despair
6. The Effects of Despair on the Body and Mind

III. Coping Strategies

1. Identifying and Managing Triggers
2. Mindfulness and Relaxation Techniques
   - Meditation
   - Progressive Muscle Relaxation (PMR)
   - Visualization
3. Time Management and Organization
4. Communication and Assertiveness Skills
5. Building a Support System

IV. Professional Help

1. When to Seek Professional Help
2. Types of Therapy
   - Cognitive Behavioral Therapy (CBT)

I.   Introduction

Introduction: A Path to Emotional Freedom and Resilience

Everybody at some point in their lives will encounter universal experiences including stress and hopelessness. The pressures of job, family, and personal goals can seem unrelenting in our fast-paced modern society, giving little time to relax, consider, or renew. Although stress is inevitable in life, when left unbridled it can develop into chronic stress and despair that seriously affects our general quality of life, mental health, and physical condition. Your road map to negotiate these obstacles with confidence, clarity, and bravery is this book.

The Purpose of This Book

Stress and hopelessness have grown widespread in the fast-paced, high-stress environment of today and impact people in all spheres of life. One can easily become overwhelmed regarding work deadlines, financial difficulties, relationship breakdowns, or just the weight of daily obligations. Stress and depression have become silent diseases invading our families, businesses, and communities in a time when increased expectations and continual connectivity rule. Whether it's a pending project deadline, financial obligations, a stressful relationship, or the aftermath of a life-changing incident, these feelings can leave you feeling helpless and overburdened.

This book was created with a clear purpose: to empower you with the knowledge, tools, and strategies needed to confront stress and despair head-on. By combining evidence-based techniques with practical advice, it provides a comprehensive roadmap to help you regain control over your emotional and mental well-being.

Through this guide, you will learn to:

- Recognize the root causes of your stress and despair.
- Understand how these emotions affect your body, mind, and relationships.
- Develop healthy habits and coping mechanisms to mitigate their impact.
- Build emotional resilience to navigate future challenges with strength and grace.

This book is not just about managing stress and despair—it's about conquering them, rediscovering joy, and creating a life of balance, purpose, and fulfillment.

What You Can Expect to Learn

To ensure a structured and effective approach, this guide is divided into five carefully designed sections. Each section addresses a critical aspect of understanding, managing, and overcoming stress and despair:

1. **Understanding Stress and Despair:**
   In the first section, you'll gain a foundational understanding of what stress and despair truly are. This includes their definitions, common causes, and the profound effects they have on your physical and mental health. By recognizing how these emotions manifest, you'll be better equipped to address them.
2. **Coping Strategies:**
   Managing stress and despair requires actionable strategies. In this section, you'll learn how to identify triggers, practice mindfulness, organize your time effectively, communicate assertively, and build a reliable support system. Each strategy is illustrated with examples to help you implement them in your daily life.
3. **Professional Help:**
   Sometimes, stress and despair exceed what can be managed through self-help alone. This section guides you on when and how to seek professional assistance. It explores therapeutic options such as Cognitive Behavioral Therapy (CBT), Dialectical Behavior Therapy (DBT), group therapy, and medications, offering insights into finding the right practitioner for your needs.
4. **Self-Care and Wellness:**
   Self-care is not a luxury—it is a necessity. This section highlights the importance of prioritizing your well-being through practices like exercise, proper nutrition, adequate sleep, and self-compassion. You'll also learn how small, consistent changes in your lifestyle can lead to significant improvements in your emotional health.
5. **Conclusion and Beyond:**
   The final section ties together the lessons learned and provides encouragement to continue your journey toward emotional wellness. It

includes additional resources, such as books, websites, and apps, to further support your progress.

By the end of this book, you'll have a well-rounded toolkit to manage stress and despair, as well as the confidence to face life's challenges with resilience and optimism.

The Impact of Stress and Despair

Stress and despair are not merely fleeting emotions—they are societal challenges with far-reaching consequences. Studies consistently reveal the pervasive impact of chronic stress on physical and mental health. According to the American Psychological Association (APA), prolonged stress can lead to:

- Increased risk of heart disease and hypertension.
- Weakening of the immune system, making individuals more susceptible to illness.
- Development of anxiety, depression, and burnout.

Often defined by emotions of hopelessness or defeat, despair can have equally terrible consequences. In severe situations, it can cause self-harm or drug misuse in addition to reducing quality of life and causing social disengagement and loss of output. For example, a World Health Organization (WHO) study shows that depression and anxiety disorders cost the world economy an estimated $1 trillion yearly in missed output.

These challenges are not confined to the individual. Stress and despair ripple outward, affecting families, workplaces, and communities. Marital conflicts, poor work performance, and strained friendships are common byproducts, underscoring the urgency of addressing these issues.

Hope and the Path Forward

There is optimism even if the numbers and narratives seem frightening. Though at times overwhelming, stress and despair are controllable with the correct information and tools. Think of the narrative of a young professional crushed under increasing deadlines and personal disappointments. By means of mindfulness techniques, counseling, and strengthening of a support system, they were able to change their life and regain resilience and joy. Their narrative reminds us that transformation is feasible—and this book will help you to reach it.

The path to emotional liberation starts with one step—that of choosing to give your health first priority. Patience, tenacity, and the direction this book provides can help you to overcome anxiety and despair, release your potential, and lead a healthy, happy life.

Let us therefore start this trip together. This book will be your friend whether your needs are for long-term answers, instant respite, or a better awareness of yourself since it will provide you with the means to flourish in the face of adversity. The good news is, though, that despair and stress are not insurmountable. You can overcome them and flourish with the correct strategy, attitude, and mindset with support.

II. Understanding Stress and Despair

What Are Stress and Despair?

Stress is a natural physiological and psychological response to challenging or threatening situations. It triggers the body's fight-or-flight response, releasing adrenaline and cortisol to help you react quickly. While short-term stress can be motivating, chronic stress becomes detrimental to health.

Despair, on the other hand, is a deep sense of hopelessness or defeat. It often arises when individuals feel trapped in situations with no clear solution or escape. Unlike stress, which can ebb and flow, despair tends to linger, affecting one's emotional and mental well-being.

Understanding Stress and Despair: Expanded Section

Common Causes of Stress and Despair

Stress

Stress arises when the demands of life exceed your perceived ability to cope. Here are some common causes of stress, along with examples:

- **Work-Related Pressures**:
  - Deadlines, performance expectations, and workplace dynamics often create significant stress. For instance, an employee managing multiple projects might feel overwhelmed by tight deadlines, resulting in burnout.
  - Job insecurity can also amplify stress, such as when a company announces layoffs, leaving employees anxious about their future.
- **Financial Struggles or Debt**:
  - Financial challenges are a common stressor. Imagine a single parent juggling bills, mortgage payments, and unexpected expenses like car repairs. The constant worry about making ends meet can take a toll on mental health.
  - For younger adults, student loan debt is a growing source of stress, often accompanied by the fear of not finding a high-paying job to offset their repayments.
- **Family Responsibilities and Conflicts**:
  - Balancing family responsibilities, such as raising children, caring for aging parents, or managing household chores, can lead to stress. For example, a middle-aged adult in the "sandwich generation" might feel torn between attending to their children's needs and supporting their elderly parents.
  - Family conflicts, such as disagreements over finances, parenting styles, or unresolved past issues, can further heighten stress levels.
- **Health Issues or Caregiving Responsibilities**:
  - Coping with a chronic illness or disability often creates stress. For instance, someone managing diabetes might feel overwhelmed by the need for constant monitoring, lifestyle changes, and medical appointments.
  - Caregiving responsibilities can also cause stress. A caregiver for a loved one with Alzheimer's might experience exhaustion, isolation, and a sense of being trapped in an unending cycle of demands.

Despair

Despair is a deep, enduring sense of hopelessness that often arises when individuals feel powerless in the face of challenges. Examples of common causes include:

- **Loss of a Loved One or Significant Life Change**:
    - Losing a spouse, parent, or close friend can plunge someone into despair, particularly if the relationship was central to their life. For instance, an elderly widow might feel lost after the death of her partner of 50 years, struggling to adjust to a life of solitude.
    - Life changes, such as divorce or losing a job, can also trigger despair. A middle-aged professional laid off after years at a company might feel they've lost their identity and purpose.
- **Chronic Illness or Physical Disability**:
    - Living with a long-term illness, such as cancer, or a physical disability can lead to despair. For example, a young athlete who becomes paralyzed after an accident may feel a profound loss of independence and identity.
    - The persistent pain or limitations caused by such conditions can make daily life feel overwhelming, contributing to a sense of hopelessness.
- **Persistent Failures or Setbacks**:
    - Repeated failures, such as being unable to pass an important exam, struggling to start a business, or facing constant rejection in job applications, can leave individuals feeling defeated and trapped in a cycle of despair.
    - For instance, an entrepreneur who invests time, energy, and savings into multiple ventures that fail might begin to question their worth and abilities.
- **Social Isolation or Lack of a Support System**:
    - Loneliness is a significant contributor to despair. A young adult who moves to a new city for work might struggle to form connections and feel increasingly isolated.
    - Those without a support system—such as immigrants who leave their families behind—may find it harder to cope with life's challenges, deepening their sense of despair.

The Effects of Stress and Despair on the Body and Mind

Stress and despair have profound and often interconnected effects on both physical health and psychological well-being.

Physical Effects

1. **Fatigue, Headaches, and Muscle Tension**:
   - Chronic stress often leaves people feeling physically drained, even after a full night's sleep. This fatigue can reduce productivity and motivation.
   - Stress-induced tension frequently manifests as headaches or neck, back, and shoulder pain, as seen in people who spend long hours at a computer without breaks.
2. **Weakened Immune System**:
   - Stress suppresses the immune system, making individuals more susceptible to illnesses. For instance, a college student facing final exams might experience recurrent colds or flu due to prolonged stress.
3. **Insomnia or Disrupted Sleep Patterns**:
   - Stress and despair often lead to sleep disturbances. A person worrying about their finances may find themselves lying awake at night, replaying the same concerns. Conversely, someone in despair might sleep excessively as a way to escape their feelings.
4. **Increased Risk of Heart Disease and Stroke**:
   - High-stress levels cause the heart to work harder, raising blood pressure and increasing the risk of cardiovascular issues. For example, individuals in high-pressure jobs may experience hypertension, a precursor to heart disease or stroke.

Psychological Effects

1. **Anxiety and Depression**:
   - Stress often fuels anxiety, with sufferers constantly anticipating the worst outcomes. For example, a young professional worried about a presentation might overthink every possible mistake, amplifying their anxiety.
   - Despair, meanwhile, often leads to depression, marked by a persistent sense of sadness and lack of interest in previously enjoyable activities. A retiree struggling to find purpose might retreat from social interactions and lose interest in hobbies.

2. **Difficulty Concentrating or Making Decisions**:
    - Stress clouds judgment and impairs focus. For instance, a college student juggling coursework and a part-time job might find it difficult to focus during lectures or retain information.
    - Despair can worsen this, leaving individuals paralyzed when faced with even simple decisions, like choosing what to eat.
3. **Irritability and Mood Swings**:
    - Stress often heightens emotional reactivity, causing minor inconveniences to trigger disproportionate anger or frustration. A parent stressed about work deadlines might snap at their children over trivial matters.
    - Despair, on the other hand, can cause erratic mood swings, ranging from apathy to outbursts of anger or grief.
4. **Feelings of Helplessness or Worthlessness**:
    - Chronic stress can erode confidence, making individuals feel incapable of handling life's demands. For example, someone consistently overlooked for promotions might start doubting their abilities.
    - Despair often amplifies these feelings, with sufferers believing they have no value or that their circumstances will never improve. A long-term unemployed individual may begin to feel like a burden to their family.

Stress and despair, while common, are complex experiences that impact all facets of life. By understanding their causes and recognizing their effects on the body and mind, individuals can take the first steps toward managing these challenging emotions and reclaiming a sense of control. Awareness is the foundation of change, and from here, we can explore strategies to heal and thrive. By understanding these effects, you can begin to recognize and address the warning signs in your own life.

III. Coping Strategies

Expanding the Toolbox for Managing Stress and Despair

When stress and despair dominate our lives, they cloud our judgment, disrupt our daily routines, and hinder our ability to thrive. Coping strategies provide the foundation for regaining control, fostering resilience, and promoting emotional well-being. This section explores practical and evidence-based approaches to manage triggers, cultivate mindfulness, and build a supportive environment.

---

1. Identifying and Managing Triggers

The cornerstone of managing stress and despair is understanding their origins. Identifying your personal triggers enables you to take proactive steps to minimize their impact.

- **Keeping a Journal:**
  Begin by maintaining a stress journal. Record situations that leave you feeling overwhelmed, your emotional responses, and the actions you took to manage the situation. For example, if you find yourself feeling stressed after meetings with a particular colleague, note the specific interactions, your thoughts, and any physical symptoms (e.g., headaches or a racing heart).
- **Analyzing Patterns:**
  Over time, your journal will reveal recurring patterns or triggers. Are your mornings consistently chaotic? Does your anxiety spike during certain times of the month, such as when bills are due? Identifying these patterns empowers you to plan and respond more effectively.
- **Implementing Changes:**
  Once you've identified triggers, take steps to avoid or better manage them. For instance, if you realize that procrastination contributes to stress, implement structured time-blocking techniques to tackle tasks incrementally. If certain relationships cause despair, consider setting boundaries or seeking professional support to navigate those dynamics.

---

2. Mindfulness and Relaxation Techniques

Mindfulness and relaxation are powerful tools for calming the mind and reducing the physiological effects of stress. These techniques promote self-awareness, helping you respond to challenges with greater clarity and composure.

- **Meditation:**
  Practicing mindfulness meditation for just 10–15 minutes a day can

significantly reduce stress levels. Find a quiet space, close your eyes, and focus on your breath. If your mind wanders, gently redirect your attention back to your breathing. For example, guided meditation apps such as Headspace or Calm can assist beginners by providing structured sessions. Regular meditation not only calms the mind but also improves focus and emotional regulation.

- **Progressive Muscle Relaxation (PMR):**
  PMR involves tensing and then relaxing each muscle group in your body, starting from your toes and working up to your head. For instance, while sitting in a chair, tense your calves for 5 seconds, then release. This technique helps release built-up physical tension caused by stress and cultivates a sense of deep relaxation.
- **Visualization:**
  Visualization, also known as guided imagery, is a mental exercise that involves imagining a peaceful and serene environment. Picture yourself on a quiet beach, with waves gently lapping the shore and the warmth of the sun on your skin. Engage your senses—hear the sound of the water, feel the sand beneath your feet. Visualization helps you mentally escape from stressful situations, creating a sense of calm even during chaos.

---

3. Time Management and Organization

Effective time management and organization are critical for reducing stress and avoiding the feeling of being overwhelmed by endless demands.

- **Prioritize Tasks:**
  Use tools like to-do lists or digital apps to prioritize your tasks based on urgency and importance. The Eisenhower Matrix, for example, categorizes tasks into four quadrants: urgent/important, not urgent/important, urgent/not important, and not urgent/not important. By focusing on high-priority tasks, you can avoid wasting energy on non-essential activities.
- **Break Down Projects:**
  Large projects can feel daunting, contributing to stress. Break them down into smaller, manageable steps. For example, instead of tackling an entire report in one sitting, set incremental goals like outlining the structure on Day 1, drafting the introduction on Day 2, and so on. This approach reduces overwhelm and ensures steady progress.

- **Set Realistic Deadlines:**
  Overcommitting often leads to stress and despair. Learn to set realistic deadlines and practice saying "no" when your plate is full. For example, if a colleague requests help with a project, assess your current commitments before agreeing. Respectfully declining when necessary protects your time and energy.

4. Communication and Assertiveness Skills

Ineffective communication often compounds stress and despair, especially when needs and boundaries are not expressed clearly. Learning to communicate assertively fosters healthier relationships and reduces unnecessary conflicts.

- **Expressing Needs and Boundaries:**
  Assertive communication involves expressing your needs, feelings, and limits respectfully but firmly. For example, if a coworker consistently interrupts your focus with non-urgent requests, you might say, "I value our collaboration, but I need uninterrupted time to complete my tasks. Could we schedule a time to discuss this later?" This approach maintains professionalism while establishing boundaries.
- **Active Listening:**
  Active listening is equally important. Focus on understanding the speaker's perspective without interrupting or formulating your response prematurely. For instance, during a disagreement with a friend, paraphrase their concerns to confirm your understanding: "So you're saying you felt ignored when I didn't respond to your message. Is that correct?" Active listening fosters empathy and reduces the likelihood of escalation.
- **Managing Conflict:**
  When conflicts arise, approach them with a problem-solving mindset rather than an adversarial attitude. For example, if a partner accuses you of neglecting household responsibilities, respond with curiosity rather than defensiveness: "I didn't realize you felt that way. How can we share these tasks more effectively?" This collaborative approach defuses tension and promotes constructive dialogue.

5. Building a Support System

No one should face stress and despair alone. A strong support system provides emotional reassurance, practical assistance, and a sense of belonging during difficult times.

- **Relying on Friends and Family:**
  Lean on trusted friends or family members for encouragement and perspective. For example, a close friend might offer valuable advice when you're navigating a career decision, or a sibling might lend a listening ear after a difficult day.
- **Joining Support Groups:**
  Sometimes, the best understanding comes from individuals with similar experiences. Join support groups, whether in-person or online, where members share strategies and offer mutual encouragement. For instance, caregivers of individuals with chronic illnesses might benefit from joining a caregiver support group, where they can exchange tips and find solace in shared experiences.
- **Seeking Mentorship:**
  In professional settings, having a mentor can alleviate stress by providing guidance and reassurance. For example, an entry-level employee overwhelmed by workplace demands might turn to a seasoned colleague for advice on navigating office culture and setting priorities.
- **Professional Networks:**
  Consider participating in professional associations or community organizations. These groups not only provide networking opportunities but also foster a sense of belonging and collective purpose. For example, a young entrepreneur could join a local business association to connect with peers and gain inspiration from shared success stories.

Final Thoughts on Coping Strategies

Though the benefits are transforming, developing good coping mechanisms calls both dedication and repetition. You may greatly lower stress and hopelessness by spotting triggers, practicing mindfulness, time management, good communication, and strong support system building. These techniques are proactive methods to help one lead a more balanced, fulfilling life rather than only reactive ones. Remember that improvement is slow as you include these methods into your daily schedule; honor little successes and keep patient with yourself. Assemble encouraging friends, relatives, or coworkers who can offer perspective and motivation. For advice and common experiences, think about visiting support groups or internet communities.

IV. Professional Help

Seeking Professional Help: A Path to Recovery

While self-help strategies can often alleviate stress and despair, there are times when professional intervention becomes essential. Recognizing the need for help and understanding the available options can empower individuals to seek timely support and achieve emotional well-being.

1. When to Seek Professional Help

Professional help is critical when stress and despair escalate to the point of interfering with one's ability to function in daily life. Some warning signs that indicate it's time to seek professional assistance include:

- **Persistent Sadness or Anxiety:**
  Feeling sad or anxious occasionally is part of life, but if these feelings persist for weeks or months without relief, they may signal an underlying mental health condition. For instance, a person who experiences unrelenting sadness and finds it difficult to enjoy activities they once loved might be struggling with clinical depression.
- **Difficulty Functioning at Work or Home:**
  Stress and despair often impair concentration, decision-making, and productivity. For example, an employee who once excelled at work may find themselves missing deadlines, avoiding tasks, or feeling overwhelmed by routine responsibilities. At home, strained relationships or neglected duties might indicate the need for professional support.
- **Suicidal Thoughts or Self-Harm Behaviors:**
  Suicidal ideation or engaging in self-harming behaviors is a serious red flag that requires immediate intervention. For example, someone experiencing

thoughts of ending their life or engaging in harmful actions such as cutting needs urgent support from a mental health professional or crisis hotline.

Seeking help early can prevent these challenges from worsening, providing individuals with the tools to manage their emotions and regain stability.

---

2. Types of Therapy

Therapy offers a structured and evidence-based approach to understanding and addressing stress and despair. Several therapeutic modalities have been proven effective:

- **Cognitive Behavioral Therapy (CBT):**
  CBT is one of the most widely used forms of therapy for managing stress, anxiety, and depression. It focuses on identifying and challenging negative thought patterns and replacing them with healthier, more constructive beliefs. For example, a person who struggles with perfectionism and feels "not good enough" might learn through CBT to reframe their thoughts, such as recognizing that mistakes are opportunities for growth rather than signs of failure.
- **Dialectical Behavior Therapy (DBT):**
  Originally developed to treat borderline personality disorder, DBT is also effective for individuals struggling with intense emotions, self-harm, or chronic despair. DBT emphasizes emotional regulation, mindfulness, and interpersonal effectiveness. For example, someone prone to emotional outbursts might use DBT techniques like deep breathing and "radical acceptance" to respond more calmly in challenging situations.
- **Group Therapy:**
  Group therapy provides a supportive environment where individuals can share their experiences and learn from others facing similar challenges. For instance, a person grieving the loss of a loved one might join a bereavement group, where they find comfort and healing in hearing others' stories and discovering they are not alone. The group dynamic fosters empathy, mutual encouragement, and a sense of belonging.
- **Trauma-Focused Therapy:**
  For those whose stress or despair stems from traumatic events, trauma-focused therapies such as Eye Movement Desensitization and Reprocessing (EMDR) or Trauma-Focused CBT can be transformative. For example, a

survivor of a car accident who experiences flashbacks and hypervigilance might work with a trauma-focused therapist to process the event and reduce the intensity of their emotional responses.

3. Medications

In some cases, therapy alone may not be enough to manage severe symptoms of stress and despair. Medications, when prescribed by a qualified healthcare professional, can help stabilize mood and reduce overwhelming feelings, allowing individuals to focus on therapy and other coping strategies.

- **Antidepressants:**
  Medications such as selective serotonin reuptake inhibitors (SSRIs) are commonly prescribed for depression and anxiety disorders. For example, someone who struggles with persistent feelings of sadness and a lack of energy might benefit from an SSRI, which can help regulate mood and restore balance to brain chemicals.
- **Anti-Anxiety Medications:**
  For those with intense anxiety or panic attacks, short-term use of anti-anxiety medications like benzodiazepines might be recommended. For example, a person with a fear of flying might use such medication temporarily to manage their symptoms before a flight. However, these medications are typically prescribed with caution due to the risk of dependence.
- **Mood Stabilizers:**
  For individuals with mood disorders such as bipolar disorder, mood stabilizers like lithium or anticonvulsants may be prescribed to manage the extreme highs and lows associated with the condition.
- **Consulting a Professional:**
  Medications should always be taken under the guidance of a licensed healthcare provider. It's important to discuss potential side effects, benefits, and risks with your doctor or psychiatrist. For example, someone prescribed an antidepressant should have regular check-ins with their provider to monitor progress and adjust the dosage if needed.

4. Finding the Right Practitioner

The effectiveness of therapy often depends on finding a practitioner who aligns with your needs and values. Consider the following factors when choosing a therapist or counselor:

- **Credentials and Expertise:**
  Ensure the practitioner is licensed and has expertise in the area you need help with. For example, someone struggling with PTSD might look for a therapist who specializes in trauma-focused therapies.
- **Compatibility and Comfort:**
  Building trust and rapport with your therapist is crucial. If you feel uncomfortable or unsupported during sessions, it's okay to seek another practitioner. For example, if you're a working professional seeking therapy for workplace stress, you might feel more comfortable with a therapist who has experience addressing career-related challenges.
- **Cultural Sensitivity:**
  Choose a practitioner who respects and understands your cultural background, values, and beliefs. For instance, a client from a religious community might seek a therapist who is sensitive to their spiritual needs and worldview.
- **Availability and Logistics:**
  Consider practical factors such as location, session frequency, and cost. Telehealth options are increasingly available, allowing individuals to access therapy remotely. For example, a busy parent might benefit from virtual sessions that fit into their schedule.
- **Evaluating the Match:**
  Therapy is a collaborative process, and it's essential to feel comfortable and supported. If you feel your therapist isn't the right fit, don't hesitate to seek another. For example, if a therapist's approach feels too rigid or unrelatable, switching to one who offers a more compassionate or personalized style could make a significant difference.

Conclusion of the Section

Seeking professional help is not a sign of weakness but an act of strength and self-care. Therapists, counselors, and psychiatrists provide the expertise and tools needed to navigate the complexities of stress and despair. Whether through therapy, medication, or a combination of both, professional intervention can offer clarity, healing, and hope. Remember, finding the right support takes time, but the journey toward emotional well-being is well worth the effort.

When to Seek Professional Help

If stress and despair begin to interfere with your daily life, relationships, or physical health, it may be time to seek professional help. Signs include:

- Persistent sadness or anxiety.
- Difficulty functioning at work or home.
- Suicidal thoughts or self-harm behaviors.

Types of Therapy

- **Cognitive Behavioral Therapy (CBT):** Helps reframe negative thoughts and develop healthier coping mechanisms.
- **Dialectical Behavior Therapy (DBT):** Focuses on emotional regulation and mindfulness.
- **Group Therapy:** Provides a supportive environment to share and learn from others.

Medications

In some cases, medications such as antidepressants or anti-anxiety drugs may be recommended to manage symptoms. Always consult a healthcare professional to discuss risks and benefits.

Finding the Right Practitioner

When choosing a therapist or counselor, consider their credentials, areas of expertise, and your personal comfort level. Don't hesitate to switch practitioners if you feel the match isn't right.

V. Self-Care and Wellness

The Role of Self-Care

Self-care is not a luxury—it's a necessity. Taking time to nurture your physical, emotional, and mental well-being is crucial for reducing stress and preventing despair.

Key Strategies for Wellness

- **Exercise:** Engage in regular physical activity, such as walking, yoga, or swimming, to boost endorphins and improve mood.
- **Nutrition:** Eat a balanced diet rich in fruits, vegetables, and lean proteins while limiting processed foods and sugar.
- **Sleep:** Prioritize 7–9 hours of quality sleep per night by maintaining a consistent schedule and creating a relaxing bedtime routine.

Self-Compassion

Treat yourself with kindness and patience. Replace self-criticism with positive affirmations and remind yourself that setbacks are a natural part of growth.

VI. Conclusion

Conclusion: A Commitment to Growth and Emotional Wellness

Stress and despair, while inevitable aspects of life, need not define your journey. This guide has provided a framework to help you better understand, manage, and overcome these difficult emotions. As we conclude, let us revisit the core lessons learned and empower you to take charge of your emotional well-being.

Key Takeaways

- **Stress and Despair Are Universal Yet Manageable:**
  Stress and despair are natural responses to life's challenges, but they don't have to dictate your actions or outlook. Recognizing these emotions as part of the human experience helps to demystify their impact and reduces feelings of isolation. For example, understanding that workplace stress is a common experience can motivate you to seek better time management tools or have open conversations with colleagues.

- **Coping Strategies Are Essential Tools for Resilience:**
  The guide emphasized actionable strategies like mindfulness, time management, and assertive communication, each designed to address the multifaceted nature of stress and despair. Implementing these strategies in daily life can yield noticeable improvements. For instance, a person struggling with financial stress might find relief by creating a realistic budget and breaking debt repayment into manageable steps, fostering both emotional and financial stability.
- **Building Resilience Takes Time:**
  Developing resilience isn't an overnight process; it's a gradual journey of small, consistent steps. Each decision to take care of yourself—whether it's practicing mindfulness, seeking professional help, or leaning on a support system—contributes to long-term emotional health. For example, starting with a five-minute daily meditation may seem small, but over weeks and months, it can significantly reduce anxiety and enhance your overall sense of control.

Encouragement to Continue

The path to reclaiming your life from stress and despair is within your reach. You've already taken a crucial step by seeking knowledge and guidance through this book. Each moment you dedicate to understanding yourself and implementing these strategies moves you closer to emotional freedom and fulfillment.

Remember, progress is not linear, and setbacks are a natural part of the journey. On days when it feels difficult, remind yourself of the resilience you've already built. For example, reflect on a past challenge you've overcome and use that as evidence of your strength and ability to grow.

You are not alone in this journey. Millions of people face similar struggles, and countless resources and support systems exist to help you navigate your unique path. Trust in the process and remain patient with yourself, knowing that every effort you make is a step toward a brighter, more balanced future.

Additional Resources for Continued Growth

As you move forward, you may find it helpful to explore additional resources to deepen your understanding and support your growth. Below are some recommendations:

- **Books to Empower and Educate:**
  - *The Stress Solution* by Dr. Rangan Chatterjee: This practical guide offers science-backed solutions for reducing stress and promoting holistic well-being, with actionable steps you can incorporate into your daily life.
  - *Feeling Good: The New Mood Therapy* by Dr. David D. Burns: A must-read for those battling negative thought patterns, this book introduces readers to Cognitive Behavioral Therapy techniques for overcoming depression and anxiety.
- **Websites for Expert Guidance:**
  - American Psychological Association (APA): A comprehensive resource for learning about stress, mental health, and evidence-based coping strategies.
  - National Alliance on Mental Illness (NAMI): An organization offering resources, support groups, and advocacy for individuals affected by mental health challenges.
- **Apps and Tools for Everyday Support:**
  - *Headspace:* A mindfulness and meditation app designed to help you reduce stress and improve focus through guided exercises.
  - *Moodfit:* A mental health fitness app that tracks your mood, offers coping strategies, and helps you identify triggers over time.

Final Words of Encouragement

You are capable of overcoming life's challenges and embracing a future filled with hope and balance. By equipping yourself with the tools outlined in this guide, you have already taken a courageous step toward reclaiming control over your emotions and well-being.

Be kind to yourself in this process. Change takes time, but every small victory—whether it's getting a full night's sleep, resolving a conflict through assertive communication, or simply feeling a bit lighter—deserves celebration.

As you continue this journey, keep this truth in mind: You are stronger than you think, and brighter days are ahead. Trust in your ability to heal, grow, and thrive, and remember that help is always available when you need it. You are never alone in this journey, and your well-being matters.

With these parting words, take the lessons you've learned and embark on the next chapter of your life with confidence and courage. Your path to a more balanced and fulfilling life begins today.

Appendix: Resources and Additional Information

This appendix serves as a comprehensive guide to further resources that can support your journey in managing and overcoming stress and despair. Whether you are seeking self-help tools, professional assistance, or community-based support, the following resources will provide valuable information and practical strategies.

I. Books and Publications

Reading can be a powerful way to expand your understanding and learn new coping techniques. Below is a curated list of books authored by mental health professionals, researchers, and personal development experts:

Stress and Emotional Management

1. **The Stress Solution** by Dr. Rangan Chatterjee
   - *Summary:* Offers actionable tips to combat stress, improve sleep, and promote relaxation. The book provides science-backed advice to simplify your life and improve well-being.
   - *Best For:* Readers seeking a holistic and practical approach to reducing stress in daily life.

2. **Burnout: The Secret to Unlocking the Stress Cycle** by Emily Nagoski and Amelia Nagoski
    - o *Summary:* Focuses on the physiological and emotional impact of stress and offers guidance on completing the stress cycle to avoid burnout.
    - o *Best For:* Professionals and caregivers experiencing chronic stress or exhaustion.
3. **Calm: Working Through Life's Daily Stresses to Find a Peaceful Center** by Dr. Arlene K. Unger
    - o *Summary:* This book provides mindfulness-based techniques to achieve calm and balance, including breathing exercises and visualizations.
    - o *Best For:* Beginners looking to integrate mindfulness into their routine.

Depression and Emotional Healing

4. **Feeling Good: The New Mood Therapy** by Dr. David D. Burns
    - o *Summary:* A foundational guide to Cognitive Behavioral Therapy (CBT) techniques for managing depression, challenging negative thoughts, and promoting optimism.
    - o *Best For:* Individuals experiencing persistent negative thoughts or low mood.
5. **The Happiness Trap** by Dr. Russ Harris
    - o *Summary:* Introduces Acceptance and Commitment Therapy (ACT) to help individuals accept difficult emotions and focus on creating a meaningful life.
    - o *Best For:* Those seeking to build resilience and embrace life's uncertainties.

II. Online Resources and Websites

Mental Health and Wellness Organizations

1. **American Psychological Association (APA):**
    - o Website: www.apa.org
    - o *What They Offer:* Articles, research findings, and tools to understand mental health challenges like stress, anxiety, and depression.
2. **National Alliance on Mental Illness (NAMI):**

- o Website: www.nami.org
- o *What They Offer:* Free resources, support groups, and educational programs for individuals affected by mental health issues.

3. Mental Health America (MHA):

- o Website: www.mhanational.org
- o *What They Offer:* Screening tools, self-help materials, and directories for local mental health services.

Mindfulness and Stress Reduction

4. Mindful:

- o Website: www.mindful.org
- o *What They Offer:* Articles and guided meditations for stress reduction and cultivating mindfulness.

5. Headspace App:

- o Website: www.headspace.com
- o *What They Offer:* A popular app offering meditation exercises, mindfulness training, and stress-relief programs.

Crisis Resources

6. Suicide & Crisis Lifeline (United States):

- o Phone: Dial 988
- o Website: 988lifeline.org
- o *What They Offer:* Immediate support for those experiencing suicidal thoughts, self-harm behaviors, or extreme emotional distress.

7. International Association for Suicide Prevention (IASP):

- o Website: www.iasp.info
- o *What They Offer:* A directory of crisis centers worldwide for those seeking help outside the U.S.

III. Support Groups and Community Networks

1. Online Support Groups

- o **SupportGroups.com:** A free platform where users can connect with others facing similar challenges, including stress, depression, and anxiety.

- o **Reddit (r/Anxiety, r/Depression):** Online communities where individuals share experiences, seek advice, and provide encouragement.

2. **In-Person Groups**
   - o **GriefShare:** Offers in-person and virtual support groups for those grieving the loss of a loved one.
   - o **Alcoholics Anonymous (AA):** For individuals managing addiction and its emotional toll, AA provides a network of peer-led meetings worldwide.

IV. Professional Help Directories

1. **Psychology Today Therapist Finder**
   - o Website: www.psychologytoday.com/us/therapists
   - o *What They Offer:* A directory of licensed therapists searchable by location, specialty, and insurance compatibility.
2. **BetterHelp (Online Counseling):**
   - o Website: www.betterhelp.com
   - o *What They Offer:* Affordable, flexible online therapy sessions with licensed professionals.
3. **Therapy for Black Girls (Inclusive Therapy):**
   - o Website: www.therapyforblackgirls.com
   - o *What They Offer:* Culturally sensitive resources and therapist directories for women of color.
4. **Open Path Collective (Low-Cost Therapy):**
   - o Website: www.openpathcollective.org
   - o *What They Offer:* Affordable therapy options for individuals and families without insurance.

V. Practical Tools and Apps

1. **Meditation and Relaxation Apps:**
   - o *Calm:* Guided meditations, sleep stories, and breathing exercises for stress reduction.
   - o *Insight Timer:* Free mindfulness meditations and relaxation music from a variety of teachers worldwide.
2. **Mood and Emotion Tracking Apps:**

- Moodpath: Tracks emotional patterns and offers tips for mental health improvement.
    - *Daylio:* A simple app for tracking moods, habits, and behaviors over time.
3. **Time Management Tools:**
    - *Todoist:* A digital planner for organizing tasks and prioritizing work.
    - *Trello:* A visual organization tool for managing projects and to-do lists.

VI. Additional Educational Resources

1. **Workshops and Courses**
    - **Coursera:** Offers courses like *The Science of Well-Being* by Yale University and *Mindfulness-Based Stress Reduction (MBSR)* by the University of Massachusetts.
    - **Udemy:** Affordable classes on emotional intelligence, mindfulness, and personal development.
2. **Podcasts:**
    - *The Happiness Lab with Dr. Laurie Santos:* Insights from psychology on cultivating happiness.
    - *Unlocking Us with Brené Brown:* Conversations about vulnerability, courage, and emotional resilience.

VII. Final Note

This appendix is meant to provide a launching pad for more in-depth research and help. Recall, conquering anxiety and hopelessness is a personal and continuous endeavor. These tools will help you construct a more balanced, contented existence. Know that aid is always just around the corner wherever you are traveling.

II.   Introduction

Introduction: A Path to Emotional Freedom and Resilience

Everybody at some point in their lives will encounter universal experiences including stress and hopelessness. The pressures of job, family, and personal goals can seem unrelenting in our fast-paced modern society, giving little time to relax, consider, or renew. Although stress is inevitable in life, when left unbridled it can develop into chronic stress and despair that seriously affects our general quality of life, mental health, and physical condition. Your road map to negotiate these obstacles with confidence, clarity, and bravery is this book.

The Purpose of This Book

Stress and hopelessness have grown widespread in the fast-paced, high-stress environment of today and impact people in all spheres of life. One can easily become overwhelmed with regard to work deadlines, financial difficulties, relationship breakdowns, or just the weight of daily obligations. Stress and depression have become silent diseases invading our families, businesses, and communities in a time when increased expectations and continual connectivity rule. Whether it's a pending project deadline, financial obligations, a stressful relationship, or the aftermath of a life-changing incident, these feelings can leave you feeling helpless and overburdened.

This book was created with a clear purpose: to empower you with the knowledge, tools, and strategies needed to confront stress and despair head-on. By combining evidence-based techniques with practical advice, it provides a comprehensive roadmap to help you regain control over your emotional and mental well-being.

Through this guide, you will learn to:

- Recognize the root causes of your stress and despair.
- Understand how these emotions affect your body, mind, and relationships.
- Develop healthy habits and coping mechanisms to mitigate their impact.
- Build emotional resilience to navigate future challenges with strength and grace.

This book is not just about managing stress and despair—it's about conquering them, rediscovering joy, and creating a life of balance, purpose, and fulfillment.

What You Can Expect to Learn

To ensure a structured and effective approach, this guide is divided into five carefully designed sections. Each section addresses a critical aspect of understanding, managing, and overcoming stress and despair:

6. **Understanding Stress and Despair:**
   In the first section, you'll gain a foundational understanding of what stress and despair truly are. This includes their definitions, common causes, and the profound effects they have on your physical and mental health. By recognizing how these emotions manifest, you'll be better equipped to address them.
7. **Coping Strategies:**
   Managing stress and despair requires actionable strategies. In this section, you'll learn how to identify triggers, practice mindfulness, organize your time effectively, communicate assertively, and build a reliable support system. Each strategy is illustrated with examples to help you implement them in your daily life.
8. **Professional Help:**
   Sometimes, stress and despair exceed what can be managed through self-help alone. This section guides you on when and how to seek professional assistance. It explores therapeutic options such as Cognitive Behavioral Therapy (CBT), Dialectical Behavior Therapy (DBT), group therapy, and medications, offering insights into finding the right practitioner for your needs.
9. **Self-Care and Wellness:**
   Self-care is not a luxury—it is a necessity. This section highlights the importance of prioritizing your well-being through practices like exercise, proper nutrition, adequate sleep, and self-compassion. You'll also learn how small, consistent changes in your lifestyle can lead to significant improvements in your emotional health.
10. **Conclusion and Beyond:**
   The final section ties together the lessons learned and provides encouragement to continue your journey toward emotional wellness. It

includes additional resources, such as books, websites, and apps, to further support your progress.

By the end of this book, you'll have a well-rounded toolkit to manage stress and despair, as well as the confidence to face life's challenges with resilience and optimism.

The Impact of Stress and Despair

Stress and despair are not merely fleeting emotions—they are societal challenges with far-reaching consequences. Studies consistently reveal the pervasive impact of chronic stress on physical and mental health. According to the American Psychological Association (APA), prolonged stress can lead to:

- Increased risk of heart disease and hypertension.
- Weakening of the immune system, making individuals more susceptible to illness.
- Development of anxiety, depression, and burnout.

Often defined by emotions of hopelessness or defeat, despair can have equally terrible consequences. In severe situations, it can cause self-harm or drug misuse in addition to reducing quality of life and causing social disengagement and loss of output. For example, a World Health Organization (WHO) study shows that depression and anxiety disorders cost the world economy an estimated $1 trillion yearly in missed output.

These challenges are not confined to the individual. Stress and despair ripple outward, affecting families, workplaces, and communities. Marital conflicts, poor work performance, and strained friendships are common byproducts, underscoring the urgency of addressing these issues.

Hope and the Path Forward

There is optimism even if the numbers and narratives seem frightening. Though at times overwhelming, stress and despair are controllable with the correct information and tools. Think of the narrative of a young professional crushed under increasing deadlines and personal disappointments. By means of mindfulness techniques, counseling, and strengthening of a support system, they were able to change their life and regain resilience and joy. Their narrative reminds us that transformation is feasible—and this book will help you to reach it.

The path to emotional liberation starts with one step—that of choosing to give your health first priority. Patience, tenacity, and the direction this book provides can help you to overcome anxiety and despair, release your potential, and lead a healthy, happy life.

Let us therefore start this trip together. This book will be your friend whether your needs are for long-term answers, instant respite, or a better awareness of yourself since it will provide you with the means to flourish in the face of adversity. The good news is, though, that despair and stress are not insurmount. You can overcome them and flourish with the correct strategy, attitude, and mindset with support.

II. Understanding Stress and Despair

What Are Stress and Despair?

Stress is a natural physiological and psychological response to challenging or threatening situations. It triggers the body's fight-or-flight response, releasing adrenaline and cortisol to help you react quickly. While short-term stress can be motivating, chronic stress becomes detrimental to health.

Despair, on the other hand, is a deep sense of hopelessness or defeat. It often arises when individuals feel trapped in situations with no clear solution or escape. Unlike stress, which can ebb and flow, despair tends to linger, affecting one's emotional and mental well-being.

Understanding Stress and Despair: Expanded Section

Common Causes of Stress and Despair

Stress

Stress arises when the demands of life exceed your perceived ability to cope. Here are some common causes of stress, along with examples:

- **Work-Related Pressures**:
  - Deadlines, performance expectations, and workplace dynamics often create significant stress. For instance, an employee managing multiple projects might feel overwhelmed by tight deadlines, resulting in burnout.
  - Job insecurity can also amplify stress, such as when a company announces layoffs, leaving employees anxious about their future.
- **Financial Struggles or Debt**:
  - Financial challenges are a common stressor. Imagine a single parent juggling bills, mortgage payments, and unexpected expenses like car repairs. The constant worry about making ends meet can take a toll on mental health.
  - For younger adults, student loan debt is a growing source of stress, often accompanied by the fear of not finding a high-paying job to offset their repayments.
- **Family Responsibilities and Conflicts**:
  - Balancing family responsibilities, such as raising children, caring for aging parents, or managing household chores, can lead to stress. For example, a middle-aged adult in the "sandwich generation" might feel torn between attending to their children's needs and supporting their elderly parents.
  - Family conflicts, such as disagreements over finances, parenting styles, or unresolved past issues, can further heighten stress levels.
- **Health Issues or Caregiving Responsibilities**:
  - Coping with a chronic illness or disability often creates stress. For instance, someone managing diabetes might feel overwhelmed by the need for constant monitoring, lifestyle changes, and medical appointments.
  - Caregiving responsibilities can also cause stress. A caregiver for a loved one with Alzheimer's might experience exhaustion, isolation, and a sense of being trapped in an unending cycle of demands.

Despair

Despair is a deep, enduring sense of hopelessness that often arises when individuals feel powerless in the face of challenges. Examples of common causes include:

- **Loss of a Loved One or Significant Life Change**:
  - Losing a spouse, parent, or close friend can plunge someone into despair, particularly if the relationship was central to their life. For instance, an elderly widow might feel lost after the death of her partner of 50 years, struggling to adjust to a life of solitude.
  - Life changes, such as divorce or losing a job, can also trigger despair. A middle-aged professional laid off after years at a company might feel they've lost their identity and purpose.
- **Chronic Illness or Physical Disability**:
  - Living with a long-term illness, such as cancer, or a physical disability can lead to despair. For example, a young athlete who becomes paralyzed after an accident may feel a profound loss of independence and identity.
  - The persistent pain or limitations caused by such conditions can make daily life feel overwhelming, contributing to a sense of hopelessness.
- **Persistent Failures or Setbacks**:
  - Repeated failures, such as being unable to pass an important exam, struggling to start a business, or facing constant rejection in job applications, can leave individuals feeling defeated and trapped in a cycle of despair.
  - For instance, an entrepreneur who invests time, energy, and savings into multiple ventures that fail might begin to question their worth and abilities.
- **Social Isolation or Lack of a Support System**:
  - Loneliness is a significant contributor to despair. A young adult who moves to a new city for work might struggle to form connections and feel increasingly isolated.
  - Those without a support system—such as immigrants who leave their families behind—may find it harder to cope with life's challenges, deepening their sense of despair.

The Effects of Stress and Despair on the Body and Mind

Stress and despair have profound and often interconnected effects on both physical health and psychological well-being.

Physical Effects

5. **Fatigue, Headaches, and Muscle Tension**:
   - Chronic stress often leaves people feeling physically drained, even after a full night's sleep. This fatigue can reduce productivity and motivation.
   - Stress-induced tension frequently manifests as headaches or neck, back, and shoulder pain, as seen in people who spend long hours at a computer without breaks.
6. **Weakened Immune System**:
   - Stress suppresses the immune system, making individuals more susceptible to illnesses. For instance, a college student facing final exams might experience recurrent colds or flu due to prolonged stress.
7. **Insomnia or Disrupted Sleep Patterns**:
   - Stress and despair often lead to sleep disturbances. A person worrying about their finances may find themselves lying awake at night, replaying the same concerns. Conversely, someone in despair might sleep excessively as a way to escape their feelings.
8. **Increased Risk of Heart Disease and Stroke**:
   - High-stress levels cause the heart to work harder, raising blood pressure and increasing the risk of cardiovascular issues. For example, individuals in high-pressure jobs may experience hypertension, a precursor to heart disease or stroke.

Psychological Effects

5. **Anxiety and Depression**:
   - Stress often fuels anxiety, with sufferers constantly anticipating the worst outcomes. For example, a young professional worried about a presentation might overthink every possible mistake, amplifying their anxiety.
   - Despair, meanwhile, often leads to depression, marked by a persistent sense of sadness and lack of interest in previously enjoyable activities. A retiree struggling to find purpose might retreat from social interactions and lose interest in hobbies.

6. **Difficulty Concentrating or Making Decisions**:
   - Stress clouds judgment and impairs focus. For instance, a college student juggling coursework and a part-time job might find it difficult to focus during lectures or retain information.
   - Despair can worsen this, leaving individuals paralyzed when faced with even simple decisions, like choosing what to eat.
7. **Irritability and Mood Swings**:
   - Stress often heightens emotional reactivity, causing minor inconveniences to trigger disproportionate anger or frustration. A parent stressed about work deadlines might snap at their children over trivial matters.
   - Despair, on the other hand, can cause erratic mood swings, ranging from apathy to outbursts of anger or grief.
8. **Feelings of Helplessness or Worthlessness**:
   - Chronic stress can erode confidence, making individuals feel incapable of handling life's demands. For example, someone consistently overlooked for promotions might start doubting their abilities.
   - Despair often amplifies these feelings, with sufferers believing they have no value or that their circumstances will never improve. A long-term unemployed individual may begin to feel like a burden to their family.

Stress and despair, while common, are complex experiences that impact all facets of life. By understanding their causes and recognizing their effects on the body and mind, individuals can take the first steps toward managing these challenging emotions and reclaiming a sense of control. Awareness is the foundation of change, and from here, we can explore strategies to heal and thrive. By understanding these effects, you can begin to recognize and address the warning signs in your own life.

III. Coping Strategies

Expanding the Toolbox for Managing Stress and Despair

When stress and despair dominate our lives, they cloud our judgment, disrupt our daily routines, and hinder our ability to thrive. Coping strategies provide the foundation for regaining control, fostering resilience, and promoting emotional well-being. This section explores practical and evidence-based approaches to manage triggers, cultivate mindfulness, and build a supportive environment.

1. Identifying and Managing Triggers

The cornerstone of managing stress and despair is understanding their origins. Identifying your personal triggers enables you to take proactive steps to minimize their impact.

- **Keeping a Journal:**
  Begin by maintaining a stress journal. Record situations that leave you feeling overwhelmed, your emotional responses, and the actions you took to manage the situation. For example, if you find yourself feeling stressed after meetings with a particular colleague, note the specific interactions, your thoughts, and any physical symptoms (e.g., headaches or a racing heart).
- **Analyzing Patterns:**
  Over time, your journal will reveal recurring patterns or triggers. Are your mornings consistently chaotic? Does your anxiety spike during certain times of the month, such as when bills are due? Identifying these patterns empowers you to plan and respond more effectively.
- **Implementing Changes:**
  Once you've identified triggers, take steps to avoid or better manage them. For instance, if you realize that procrastination contributes to stress, implement structured time-blocking techniques to tackle tasks incrementally. If certain relationships cause despair, consider setting boundaries or seeking professional support to navigate those dynamics.

2. Mindfulness and Relaxation Techniques

Mindfulness and relaxation are powerful tools for calming the mind and reducing the physiological effects of stress. These techniques promote self-awareness, helping you respond to challenges with greater clarity and composure.

- **Meditation:**
  Practicing mindfulness meditation for just 10–15 minutes a day can

significantly reduce stress levels. Find a quiet space, close your eyes, and focus on your breath. If your mind wanders, gently redirect your attention back to your breathing. For example, guided meditation apps such as Headspace or Calm can assist beginners by providing structured sessions. Regular meditation not only calms the mind but also improves focus and emotional regulation.

- **Progressive Muscle Relaxation (PMR):**
  PMR involves tensing and then relaxing each muscle group in your body, starting from your toes and working up to your head. For instance, while sitting in a chair, tense your calves for 5 seconds, then release. This technique helps release built-up physical tension caused by stress and cultivates a sense of deep relaxation.
- **Visualization:**
  Visualization, also known as guided imagery, is a mental exercise that involves imagining a peaceful and serene environment. Picture yourself on a quiet beach, with waves gently lapping the shore and the warmth of the sun on your skin. Engage your senses—hear the sound of the water, feel the sand beneath your feet. Visualization helps you mentally escape from stressful situations, creating a sense of calm even during chaos.

---

3. Time Management and Organization

Effective time management and organization are critical for reducing stress and avoiding the feeling of being overwhelmed by endless demands.

- **Prioritize Tasks:**
  Use tools like to-do lists or digital apps to prioritize your tasks based on urgency and importance. The Eisenhower Matrix, for example, categorizes tasks into four quadrants: urgent/important, not urgent/important, urgent/not important, and not urgent/not important. By focusing on high-priority tasks, you can avoid wasting energy on non-essential activities.
- **Break Down Projects:**
  Large projects can feel daunting, contributing to stress. Break them down into smaller, manageable steps. For example, instead of tackling an entire report in one sitting, set incremental goals like outlining the structure on Day 1, drafting the introduction on Day 2, and so on. This approach reduces overwhelm and ensures steady progress.

- **Set Realistic Deadlines:**
  Overcommitting often leads to stress and despair. Learn to set realistic deadlines and practice saying "no" when your plate is full. For example, if a colleague requests help with a project, assess your current commitments before agreeing. Respectfully declining when necessary protects your time and energy.

4. Communication and Assertiveness Skills

Ineffective communication often compounds stress and despair, especially when needs and boundaries are not expressed clearly. Learning to communicate assertively fosters healthier relationships and reduces unnecessary conflicts.

- **Expressing Needs and Boundaries:**
  Assertive communication involves expressing your needs, feelings, and limits respectfully but firmly. For example, if a coworker consistently interrupts your focus with non-urgent requests, you might say, "I value our collaboration, but I need uninterrupted time to complete my tasks. Could we schedule a time to discuss this later?" This approach maintains professionalism while establishing boundaries.
- **Active Listening:**
  Active listening is equally important. Focus on understanding the speaker's perspective without interrupting or formulating your response prematurely. For instance, during a disagreement with a friend, paraphrase their concerns to confirm your understanding: "So you're saying you felt ignored when I didn't respond to your message. Is that correct?" Active listening fosters empathy and reduces the likelihood of escalation.
- **Managing Conflict:**
  When conflicts arise, approach them with a problem-solving mindset rather than an adversarial attitude. For example, if a partner accuses you of neglecting household responsibilities, respond with curiosity rather than defensiveness: "I didn't realize you felt that way. How can we share these tasks more effectively?" This collaborative approach defuses tension and promotes constructive dialogue.

5. Building a Support System

No one should face stress and despair alone. A strong support system provides emotional reassurance, practical assistance, and a sense of belonging during difficult times.

- **Relying on Friends and Family:**
  Lean on trusted friends or family members for encouragement and perspective. For example, a close friend might offer valuable advice when you're navigating a career decision, or a sibling might lend a listening ear after a difficult day.
- **Joining Support Groups:**
  Sometimes, the best understanding comes from individuals with similar experiences. Join support groups, whether in-person or online, where members share strategies and offer mutual encouragement. For instance, caregivers of individuals with chronic illnesses might benefit from joining a caregiver support group, where they can exchange tips and find solace in shared experiences.
- **Seeking Mentorship:**
  In professional settings, having a mentor can alleviate stress by providing guidance and reassurance. For example, an entry-level employee overwhelmed by workplace demands might turn to a seasoned colleague for advice on navigating office culture and setting priorities.
- **Professional Networks:**
  Consider participating in professional associations or community organizations. These groups not only provide networking opportunities but also foster a sense of belonging and collective purpose. For example, a young entrepreneur could join a local business association to connect with peers and gain inspiration from shared success stories.

Final Thoughts on Coping Strategies

Though the benefits are transforming, developing good coping mechanisms calls both dedication and repetition. You may greatly lower stress and hopelessness by spotting triggers, practicing mindfulness, time management, good communication, and strong support system building. These techniques are proactive methods to help one lead a more balanced, fulfilling life rather than only reactive ones. Remember that improvement is slow as you include these methods into your daily schedule; honor little successes and keep patient with yourself. Assemble encouraging friends, relatives, or coworkers who can offer perspective and motivation. For advice and common experiences, think about visiting support groups or internet communities.

IV. Professional Help

Seeking Professional Help: A Path to Recovery

While self-help strategies can often alleviate stress and despair, there are times when professional intervention becomes essential. Recognizing the need for help and understanding the available options can empower individuals to seek timely support and achieve emotional well-being.

---

1. When to Seek Professional Help

Professional help is critical when stress and despair escalate to the point of interfering with one's ability to function in daily life. Some warning signs that indicate it's time to seek professional assistance include:

- **Persistent Sadness or Anxiety:**
  Feeling sad or anxious occasionally is part of life, but if these feelings persist for weeks or months without relief, they may signal an underlying mental health condition. For instance, a person who experiences unrelenting sadness and finds it difficult to enjoy activities they once loved might be struggling with clinical depression.
- **Difficulty Functioning at Work or Home:**
  Stress and despair often impair concentration, decision-making, and productivity. For example, an employee who once excelled at work may find themselves missing deadlines, avoiding tasks, or feeling overwhelmed by routine responsibilities. At home, strained relationships or neglected duties might indicate the need for professional support.
- **Suicidal Thoughts or Self-Harm Behaviors:**
  Suicidal ideation or engaging in self-harming behaviors is a serious red flag that requires immediate intervention. For example, someone experiencing

thoughts of ending their life or engaging in harmful actions such as cutting needs urgent support from a mental health professional or crisis hotline.

Seeking help early can prevent these challenges from worsening, providing individuals with the tools to manage their emotions and regain stability.

---

2. Types of Therapy

Therapy offers a structured and evidence-based approach to understanding and addressing stress and despair. Several therapeutic modalities have been proven effective:

- **Cognitive Behavioral Therapy (CBT):**
  CBT is one of the most widely used forms of therapy for managing stress, anxiety, and depression. It focuses on identifying and challenging negative thought patterns and replacing them with healthier, more constructive beliefs. For example, a person who struggles with perfectionism and feels "not good enough" might learn through CBT to reframe their thoughts, such as recognizing that mistakes are opportunities for growth rather than signs of failure.
- **Dialectical Behavior Therapy (DBT):**
  Originally developed to treat borderline personality disorder, DBT is also effective for individuals struggling with intense emotions, self-harm, or chronic despair. DBT emphasizes emotional regulation, mindfulness, and interpersonal effectiveness. For example, someone prone to emotional outbursts might use DBT techniques like deep breathing and "radical acceptance" to respond more calmly in challenging situations.
- **Group Therapy:**
  Group therapy provides a supportive environment where individuals can share their experiences and learn from others facing similar challenges. For instance, a person grieving the loss of a loved one might join a bereavement group, where they find comfort and healing in hearing others' stories and discovering they are not alone. The group dynamic fosters empathy, mutual encouragement, and a sense of belonging.
- **Trauma-Focused Therapy:**
  For those whose stress or despair stems from traumatic events, trauma-focused therapies such as Eye Movement Desensitization and Reprocessing (EMDR) or Trauma-Focused CBT can be transformative. For example, a

survivor of a car accident who experiences flashbacks and hypervigilance might work with a trauma-focused therapist to process the event and reduce the intensity of their emotional responses.

3. Medications

In some cases, therapy alone may not be enough to manage severe symptoms of stress and despair. Medications, when prescribed by a qualified healthcare professional, can help stabilize mood and reduce overwhelming feelings, allowing individuals to focus on therapy and other coping strategies.

- **Antidepressants:**
  Medications such as selective serotonin reuptake inhibitors (SSRIs) are commonly prescribed for depression and anxiety disorders. For example, someone who struggles with persistent feelings of sadness and a lack of energy might benefit from an SSRI, which can help regulate mood and restore balance to brain chemicals.
- **Anti-Anxiety Medications:**
  For those with intense anxiety or panic attacks, short-term use of anti-anxiety medications like benzodiazepines might be recommended. For example, a person with a fear of flying might use such medication temporarily to manage their symptoms before a flight. However, these medications are typically prescribed with caution due to the risk of dependence.
- **Mood Stabilizers:**
  For individuals with mood disorders such as bipolar disorder, mood stabilizers like lithium or anticonvulsants may be prescribed to manage the extreme highs and lows associated with the condition.
- **Consulting a Professional:**
  Medications should always be taken under the guidance of a licensed healthcare provider. It's important to discuss potential side effects, benefits, and risks with your doctor or psychiatrist. For example, someone prescribed an antidepressant should have regular check-ins with their provider to monitor progress and adjust the dosage if needed.

4. Finding the Right Practitioner

The effectiveness of therapy often depends on finding a practitioner who aligns with your needs and values. Consider the following factors when choosing a therapist or counselor:

- **Credentials and Expertise:**
  Ensure the practitioner is licensed and has expertise in the area you need help with. For example, someone struggling with PTSD might look for a therapist who specializes in trauma-focused therapies.
- **Compatibility and Comfort:**
  Building trust and rapport with your therapist is crucial. If you feel uncomfortable or unsupported during sessions, it's okay to seek another practitioner. For example, if you're a working professional seeking therapy for workplace stress, you might feel more comfortable with a therapist who has experience addressing career-related challenges.
- **Cultural Sensitivity:**
  Choose a practitioner who respects and understands your cultural background, values, and beliefs. For instance, a client from a religious community might seek a therapist who is sensitive to their spiritual needs and worldview.
- **Availability and Logistics:**
  Consider practical factors such as location, session frequency, and cost. Telehealth options are increasingly available, allowing individuals to access therapy remotely. For example, a busy parent might benefit from virtual sessions that fit into their schedule.
- **Evaluating the Match:**
  Therapy is a collaborative process, and it's essential to feel comfortable and supported. If you feel your therapist isn't the right fit, don't hesitate to seek another. For example, if a therapist's approach feels too rigid or unrelatable, switching to one who offers a more compassionate or personalized style could make a significant difference.

Conclusion of the Section

Seeking professional help is not a sign of weakness but an act of strength and self-care. Therapists, counselors, and psychiatrists provide the expertise and tools needed to navigate the complexities of stress and despair. Whether through therapy, medication, or a combination of both, professional intervention can offer clarity, healing, and hope. Remember, finding the right support takes time, but the journey toward emotional well-being is well worth the effort.

When to Seek Professional Help

If stress and despair begin to interfere with your daily life, relationships, or physical health, it may be time to seek professional help. Signs include:

- Persistent sadness or anxiety.
- Difficulty functioning at work or home.
- Suicidal thoughts or self-harm behaviors.

Types of Therapy

- **Cognitive Behavioral Therapy (CBT):** Helps reframe negative thoughts and develop healthier coping mechanisms.
- **Dialectical Behavior Therapy (DBT):** Focuses on emotional regulation and mindfulness.
- **Group Therapy:** Provides a supportive environment to share and learn from others.

Medications

In some cases, medications such as antidepressants or anti-anxiety drugs may be recommended to manage symptoms. Always consult a healthcare professional to discuss risks and benefits.

Finding the Right Practitioner

When choosing a therapist or counselor, consider their credentials, areas of expertise, and your personal comfort level. Don't hesitate to switch practitioners if you feel the match isn't right.

V. Self-Care and Wellness

The Role of Self-Care

Self-care is not a luxury—it's a necessity. Taking time to nurture your physical, emotional, and mental well-being is crucial for reducing stress and preventing despair.

Key Strategies for Wellness

- **Exercise:** Engage in regular physical activity, such as walking, yoga, or swimming, to boost endorphins and improve mood.
- **Nutrition:** Eat a balanced diet rich in fruits, vegetables, and lean proteins while limiting processed foods and sugar.
- **Sleep:** Prioritize 7–9 hours of quality sleep per night by maintaining a consistent schedule and creating a relaxing bedtime routine.

Self-Compassion

Treat yourself with kindness and patience. Replace self-criticism with positive affirmations and remind yourself that setbacks are a natural part of growth.

VI. Conclusion

Conclusion: A Commitment to Growth and Emotional Wellness

Stress and despair, while inevitable aspects of life, need not define your journey. This guide has provided a framework to help you better understand, manage, and overcome these difficult emotions. As we conclude, let us revisit the core lessons learned and empower you to take charge of your emotional well-being.

Key Takeaways

- **Stress and Despair Are Universal Yet Manageable:**
  Stress and despair are natural responses to life's challenges, but they don't have to dictate your actions or outlook. Recognizing these emotions as part of the human experience helps to demystify their impact and reduces feelings of isolation. For example, understanding that workplace stress is a common experience can motivate you to seek better time management tools or have open conversations with colleagues.

- **Coping Strategies Are Essential Tools for Resilience:**
  The guide emphasized actionable strategies like mindfulness, time management, and assertive communication, each designed to address the multifaceted nature of stress and despair. Implementing these strategies in daily life can yield noticeable improvements. For instance, a person struggling with financial stress might find relief by creating a realistic budget and breaking debt repayment into manageable steps, fostering both emotional and financial stability.
- **Building Resilience Takes Time:**
  Developing resilience isn't an overnight process; it's a gradual journey of small, consistent steps. Each decision to take care of yourself—whether it's practicing mindfulness, seeking professional help, or leaning on a support system—contributes to long-term emotional health. For example, starting with a five-minute daily meditation may seem small, but over weeks and months, it can significantly reduce anxiety and enhance your overall sense of control.

Encouragement to Continue

The path to reclaiming your life from stress and despair is within your reach. You've already taken a crucial step by seeking knowledge and guidance through this book. Each moment you dedicate to understanding yourself and implementing these strategies moves you closer to emotional freedom and fulfillment.

Remember, progress is not linear, and setbacks are a natural part of the journey. On days when it feels difficult, remind yourself of the resilience you've already built. For example, reflect on a past challenge you've overcome and use that as evidence of your strength and ability to grow.

You are not alone in this journey. Millions of people face similar struggles, and countless resources and support systems exist to help you navigate your unique path. Trust in the process and remain patient with yourself, knowing that every effort you make is a step toward a brighter, more balanced future.

Additional Resources for Continued Growth

As you move forward, you may find it helpful to explore additional resources to deepen your understanding and support your growth. Below are some recommendations:

- **Books to Empower and Educate:**
  - *The Stress Solution* by Dr. Rangan Chatterjee: This practical guide offers science-backed solutions for reducing stress and promoting holistic well-being, with actionable steps you can incorporate into your daily life.
  - *Feeling Good: The New Mood Therapy* by Dr. David D. Burns: A must-read for those battling negative thought patterns, this book introduces readers to Cognitive Behavioral Therapy techniques for overcoming depression and anxiety.
- **Websites for Expert Guidance:**
  - American Psychological Association (APA): A comprehensive resource for learning about stress, mental health, and evidence-based coping strategies.
  - National Alliance on Mental Illness (NAMI): An organization offering resources, support groups, and advocacy for individuals affected by mental health challenges.
- **Apps and Tools for Everyday Support:**
  - *Headspace:* A mindfulness and meditation app designed to help you reduce stress and improve focus through guided exercises.
  - *Moodfit:* A mental health fitness app that tracks your mood, offers coping strategies, and helps you identify triggers over time.

Final Words of Encouragement

You are capable of overcoming life's challenges and embracing a future filled with hope and balance. By equipping yourself with the tools outlined in this guide, you have already taken a courageous step toward reclaiming control over your emotions and well-being.

Be kind to yourself in this process. Change takes time, but every small victory—whether it's getting a full night's sleep, resolving a conflict through assertive communication, or simply feeling a bit lighter—deserves celebration.

As you continue this journey, keep this truth in mind: You are stronger than you think, and brighter days are ahead. Trust in your ability to heal, grow, and thrive, and remember that help is always available when you need it. You are never alone in this journey, and your well-being matters.

With these parting words, take the lessons you've learned and embark on the next chapter of your life with confidence and courage. Your path to a more balanced and fulfilling life begins today.

Appendix: Resources and Additional Information

This appendix serves as a comprehensive guide to further resources that can support your journey in managing and overcoming stress and despair. Whether you are seeking self-help tools, professional assistance, or community-based support, the following resources will provide valuable information and practical strategies.

I. Books and Publications

Reading can be a powerful way to expand your understanding and learn new coping techniques. Below is a curated list of books authored by mental health professionals, researchers, and personal development experts:

Stress and Emotional Management

4. **The Stress Solution** by Dr. Rangan Chatterjee
   - *Summary:* Offers actionable tips to combat stress, improve sleep, and promote relaxation. The book provides science-backed advice to simplify your life and improve well-being.
   - *Best For:* Readers seeking a holistic and practical approach to reducing stress in daily life.

5. **Burnout: The Secret to Unlocking the Stress Cycle** by Emily Nagoski and Amelia Nagoski
    o *Summary:* Focuses on the physiological and emotional impact of stress and offers guidance on completing the stress cycle to avoid burnout.
    o *Best For:* Professionals and caregivers experiencing chronic stress or exhaustion.
6. **Calm: Working Through Life's Daily Stresses to Find a Peaceful Center** by Dr. Arlene K. Unger
    o *Summary:* This book provides mindfulness-based techniques to achieve calm and balance, including breathing exercises and visualizations.
    o *Best For:* Beginners looking to integrate mindfulness into their routine.

Depression and Emotional Healing

6. **Feeling Good: The New Mood Therapy** by Dr. David D. Burns
    o *Summary:* A foundational guide to Cognitive Behavioral Therapy (CBT) techniques for managing depression, challenging negative thoughts, and promoting optimism.
    o *Best For:* Individuals experiencing persistent negative thoughts or low mood.
7. **The Happiness Trap** by Dr. Russ Harris
    o *Summary:* Introduces Acceptance and Commitment Therapy (ACT) to help individuals accept difficult emotions and focus on creating a meaningful life.
    o *Best For:* Those seeking to build resilience and embrace life's uncertainties.

II. Online Resources and Websites

Mental Health and Wellness Organizations

4. **American Psychological Association (APA):**
    o Website: www.apa.org
    o *What They Offer:* Articles, research findings, and tools to understand mental health challenges like stress, anxiety, and depression.
5. **National Alliance on Mental Illness (NAMI):**

- o Website: www.nami.org
- o *What They Offer:* Free resources, support groups, and educational programs for individuals affected by mental health issues.

6. **Mental Health America (MHA):**
   - o Website: www.mhanational.org
   - o *What They Offer:* Screening tools, self-help materials, and directories for local mental health services.

Mindfulness and Stress Reduction

6. **Mindful:**
   - o Website: www.mindful.org
   - o *What They Offer:* Articles and guided meditations for stress reduction and cultivating mindfulness.
7. **Headspace App:**
   - o Website: www.headspace.com
   - o *What They Offer:* A popular app offering meditation exercises, mindfulness training, and stress-relief programs.

Crisis Resources

8. **Suicide & Crisis Lifeline (United States):**
   - o Phone: Dial 988
   - o Website: 988lifeline.org
   - o *What They Offer:* Immediate support for those experiencing suicidal thoughts, self-harm behaviors, or extreme emotional distress.
9. **International Association for Suicide Prevention (IASP):**
   - o Website: www.iasp.info
   - o *What They Offer:* A directory of crisis centers worldwide for those seeking help outside the U.S.

III. Support Groups and Community Networks

3. **Online Support Groups**
   - o **SupportGroups.com:** A free platform where users can connect with others facing similar challenges, including stress, depression, and anxiety.

- o **Reddit (r/Anxiety, r/Depression):** Online communities where individuals share experiences, seek advice, and provide encouragement.
4. **In-Person Groups**
   - o **GriefShare:** Offers in-person and virtual support groups for those grieving the loss of a loved one.
   - o **Alcoholics Anonymous (AA):** For individuals managing addiction and its emotional toll, AA provides a network of peer-led meetings worldwide.

IV. Professional Help Directories

5. **Psychology Today Therapist Finder**
   - o Website: www.psychologytoday.com/us/therapists
   - o *What They Offer:* A directory of licensed therapists searchable by location, specialty, and insurance compatibility.
6. **BetterHelp (Online Counseling):**
   - o Website: www.betterhelp.com
   - o *What They Offer:* Affordable, flexible online therapy sessions with licensed professionals.
7. **Therapy for Black Girls (Inclusive Therapy):**
   - o Website: www.therapyforblackgirls.com
   - o *What They Offer:* Culturally sensitive resources and therapist directories for women of color.
8. **Open Path Collective (Low-Cost Therapy):**
   - o Website: www.openpathcollective.org
   - o *What They Offer:* Affordable therapy options for individuals and families without insurance.

V. Practical Tools and Apps

4. **Meditation and Relaxation Apps:**
   - o *Calm:* Guided meditations, sleep stories, and breathing exercises for stress reduction.
   - o *Insight Timer:* Free mindfulness meditations and relaxation music from a variety of teachers worldwide.
5. **Mood and Emotion Tracking Apps:**

- - *Moodpath:* Tracks emotional patterns and offers tips for mental health improvement.
    - *Daylio:* A simple app for tracking moods, habits, and behaviors over time.
6. **Time Management Tools:**
    - *Todoist:* A digital planner for organizing tasks and prioritizing work.
    - *Trello:* A visual organization tool for managing projects and to-do lists.

VI. Additional Educational Resources

3. **Workshops and Courses**
    - **Coursera:** Offers courses like *The Science of Well-Being* by Yale University and *Mindfulness-Based Stress Reduction (MBSR)* by the University of Massachusetts.
    - **Udemy:** Affordable classes on emotional intelligence, mindfulness, and personal development.
4. **Podcasts:**
    - *The Happiness Lab with Dr. Laurie Santos:* Insights from psychology on cultivating happiness.
    - *Unlocking Us with Brené Brown:* Conversations about vulnerability, courage, and emotional resilience.

VII. Final Note

This appendix is meant to provide a launching pad for more in-depth research and help. Recall, conquering anxiety and hopelessness is a personal and continuous endeavor. These tools will help you construct a more balanced, contented existence. Know that aid is always just around the corner wherever you are traveling.